M000208795

getting gorgeous

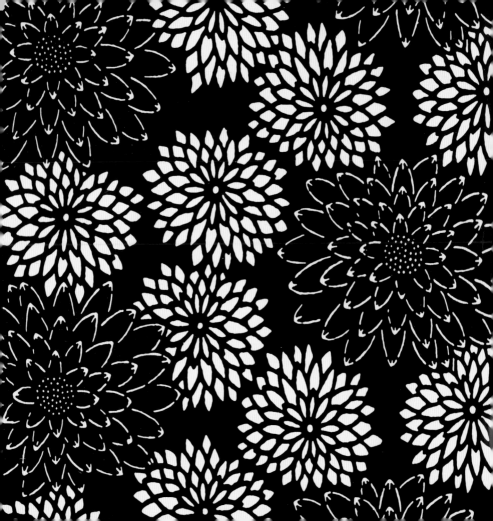

getting gorgeous

HOW TO LOOK AND FEEL FABULOUS

Jacqui Ripley

RYLAND
PETERS
& SMALL

LONDON NEW YORK

Senior Designer Amy Trombat
Commissioning Editor Annabel Morgan
Picture Researcher Jess Walton
Production Manager Patricia Harrington
Publishing Director Alison Starling

First published in the United States
in 2007 by Ryland Peters & Small, Inc
519 Broadway, 5th Floor
New York, NY 10012
www.rylandpeters.com

10 9 8 7 6 5 4 3 2 1

Text © Jacqui Ripley 2007
Design and photographs
© Ryland Peters & Small 2007

ISBN-10: 1-84597-508-1
ISBN-13: 978-1-84597-508-1

Printed in China

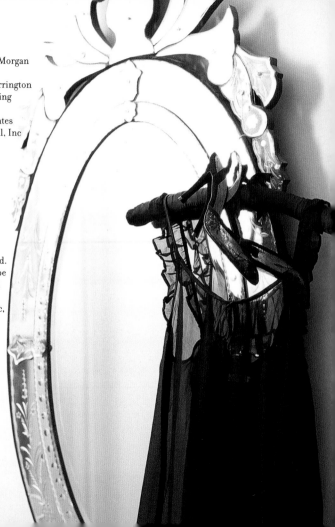

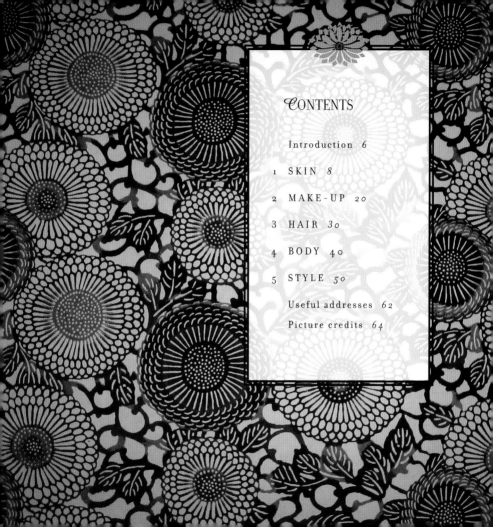

CONTENTS

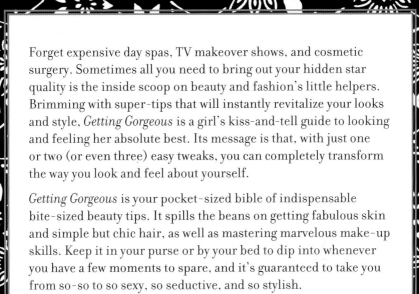

Forget expensive day spas, TV makeover shows, and cosmetic surgery. Sometimes all you need to bring out your hidden star quality is the inside scoop on beauty and fashion's little helpers. Brimming with super-tips that will instantly revitalize your looks and style, *Getting Gorgeous* is a girl's kiss-and-tell guide to looking and feeling her absolute best. Its message is that, with just one or two (or even three) easy tweaks, you can completely transform the way you look and feel about yourself.

Getting Gorgeous is your pocket-sized bible of indispensable bite-sized beauty tips. It spills the beans on getting fabulous skin and simple but chic hair, as well as mastering marvelous make-up skills. Keep it in your purse or by your bed to dip into whenever you have a few moments to spare, and it's guaranteed to take you from so-so to so sexy, so seductive, and so stylish.

Warning—only read this book if you want to feel more attractive, more irresistible, and most of all, more gorgeous!

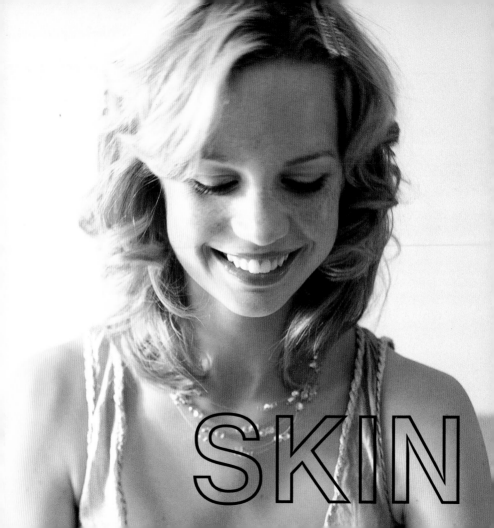

RADIANT. GLOWING. *Luminous.*

What's the secret to getting that *head-over-heels-in-love* glow to your skin? A successful skincare regimen doesn't have to be complicated—you just need to put in a little time and effort. Women with *beautiful* complexions see results because they go the extra *beauty* mile.

All too often, modern-day skincare demands cosmetic procedures that promise to restore a *youthful glow*. But get up close and personal with your skin and you will start to understand it better. Soon skin will begin to improve and take on a *natural brilliance*.

For more *good-skin days* starting right now, here are invaluable skin tips that give *instant gratification* and promise long-lasting results. Try them, and enjoy the feel and look of a clear, *radiant* complexion.

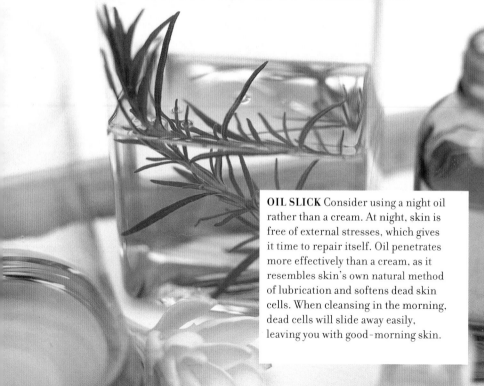

GREAT SKIN MADE SIMPLE

OIL SLICK Consider using a night oil rather than a cream. At night, skin is free of external stresses, which gives it time to repair itself. Oil penetrates more effectively than a cream, as it resembles skin's own natural method of lubrication and softens dead skin cells. When cleansing in the morning, dead cells will slide away easily, leaving you with good-morning skin.

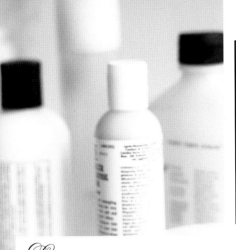

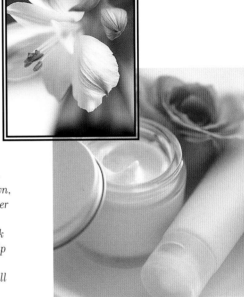

*ℒ*IGHTEN AND *BRIGHTEN* From *your mid-twenties on, cell turnover slows down, causing dead cells to collect and clump together on the skin's surface. The result? Skin reflects light more unevenly, and skin can start to look dull and dingy. Refresh your skin with the help of a microdermabrasion treatment (the latest news in exfoliation) to optimize your skin's cell renewal process. Then follow with a radiance reviver. This two-step skin trick not only leaves skin gleaming, but also allows your make-up to glide on like a dream.*

SCENT SEDUCTION Pick creams that you love the smell of (especially night creams or oils). They will then always feel like an indulgence and be a pleasure to use.

SAVE YOUR NECK The neck lacks sebaceous glands, which is why, if it's not cared for, it can look dry and lined years before your face. There's little beauty sense in lavishing attention on your face but not your neck, so always bring your skincare—including exfoliants and masks—down below your jaw line. When moisturizing, smooth your cream from the jaw all the way down to your collarbone.

OXYGENATE TO RADIATE Always open a small window at night. Sleeping in a stuffy atmosphere starves the skin of oxygen and results in a puffy, dehydrated face.

TEST YOUR EYES It's hard to stop wrinkles becoming deeper when skin is constantly folding. If you find yourself squinting frequently, get your eyes tested and, if necessary, wear glasses to ward off crow's feet!

PINCH AND POUT For plumper lips without the collagen injections, gently pinch the lip line with your thumb and forefinger, pressing in and out several times before slicking on your favorite lipstick.

EYE REVIVAL Under-eye puffiness can be due to heavy-handed application of eye cream. Don't slather it on! Instead, use the pad of your ring finger to pick up a pea-sized amount and delicately massage in a circular motion across the lid and underneath the eye.

STRIP A pore strip can be a girl's best friend. Use in between visits to your facialist to purge your nose or chin of blackheads.

WARM UP A MASK In winter, when skin craves extra comfort, pop your favorite face mask in the microwave for 30 seconds, then smooth onto your complexion for a nurturing treat. Match your masks to your skin type. Double up by using a moisturizing mask to soothe dry cheeks, and a clay mask to absorb oil on your T-zone.

BE SPF SMART Wrinkles take years to develop, and you can make them wait a little longer by shopping for a moisturizer or foundation with the inclusion of an SPF.

SKIN SLICK Save your skin with silicone. When you find yourself in an environment that's drier than the Sahara, use a face cream with generous levels of silicone. It forms a barrier on the skin to halt moisture loss, as well as making your skin look plumper and smoother.

SEASON YOUR SKIN Rotate your skincare to suit the seasons—opt for lighter formulations in the summer, when heat equals oiliness, then choose richer formulations in the winter months, when skin craves moisture. Central heating also saps skin of much-needed moisture, so either invest in some green plants that give out oxygen, or buy a large bowl, fill it with water, and place near a radiator. You can even put a couple of floating candles in to pretty it up.

AVOID STEAM Although facial steaming is often recommended, it can actually dehydrate the skin if you're prone to dryness, causing fine lines to appear. Instead, soak a washcloth in a bowl of warm water along with a couple of drops of lavender oil, squeeze it out, and place over your face to de-stress, detoxify, and relax your skin.

BE PASSIVE, NOT AGGRESSIVE

When it comes to seeking the fountain of youth, it seems everybody demands instant results to the point where the skin can become overloaded with too many potent, chemical, age-defying products. Be warned: irritation and prematurely aged skin are closely linked. Introduce new skincare products one step at a time, giving your skin enough time to adjust.

SKIN O'CLOCK

If you want to impress someone special, arrange to meet them at 2 P.M. This is the time you naturally look your best: skin color will be perky, as you're not yet fatigued (that comes at 4 P.M.!) and you literally radiate from within, as skin is full of moisture but not yet producing too much oil.

FEEL WITH FINGERTIPS

Skin needs love and affection to perform well. Sluggish skin is more prone to folding and sagging, so carry out a firming massage for at least one minute when you're applying your creams or oils. Caress the skin using even pressure—this will increase the blood flow to the surface and help to drain the skin of toxins. If you have small blemishes, facial massage will also help break those down and get rid of them faster. It's also incredibly relaxing!

FIND A FACIALIST

A great facialist can do for your skin what a talented stylist can do for your hair. Book in every six weeks for a fix-all facial that will leave skin deeply cleansed and dewy. The best facials always include an extraction and should be tailor-made to meet your skin's individual needs.

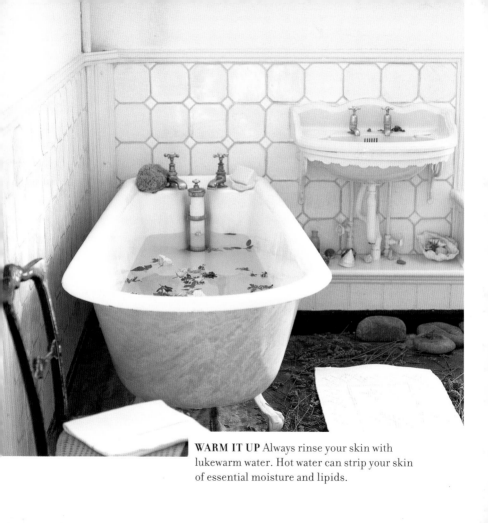

WARM IT UP Always rinse your skin with lukewarm water. Hot water can strip your skin of essential moisture and lipids.

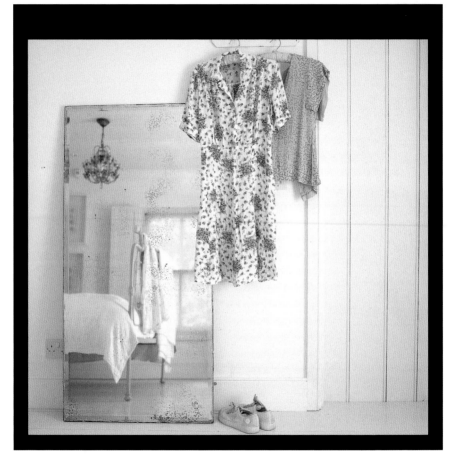

PILLOW TALK No clear-skinned beauty ever goes to bed with a dirty face. Sleeping in foundation congests the pores and turns skin sallow. However tired you are, always make time to cleanse. If you're a party girl, keep a pack of cleansing wipes beside your bed for a last minute face-off.

PARTY-PROOF SKIN Keep skin looking livelier after a night out on the town by alternating cocktails with glasses of nonsparkling water. Continual hydration saves your face from that morning-after puffiness.

STAY OFF SUGAR It's been revealed by leading skin experts that sugar not only rots teeth but ages the skin prematurely, too. Here's the science: excess sugar can bond itself to proteins in the skin in a process called glycation. This leads to skin becoming stiff, inflexible, and prone to wrinkles.

FEED WITH FATS No, not fries, but Omega 3 fatty acids! They're one of the top skin-boosting nutrients and help by modifying the production of hormones that encourage healing and control tissue growth. Find them in oily fish such as mackerel or salmon. Be warned that hydrogenated fats—found in mass-produced cookies and cakes—have the reverse effect. They can unbalance your hormonal system, which in turn can give rise to troublesome skin.

DRINK ORGANIC If drinking wine leaves your cheeks flushed, then sip organic—it has fewer skin reddening chemical additives.

CHILL AND REVIVE Keep both your eye make-up remover and daily moisturizer in the fridge. The initial coolness will stimulate the skin—as well as other senses—and help reduce congestion.

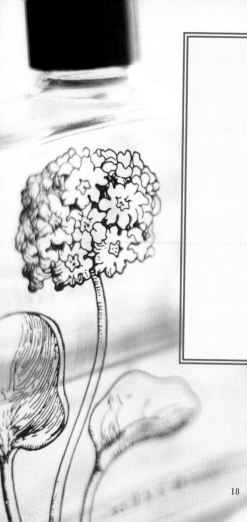

CLEAN BEFORE TONING Cleanse before you hit the gym. A combination of moisturizer and foundation can form a barrier on the skin that blocks the evaporation of sweat, which can quickly result in blemishes.

SWIPE AWAY BREAKOUTS Your phone can be the cause of unwanted outbreaks around the chin, mouth, and temples—not very glamorous! Regularly clean your handset with a cleansing or antibacterial wipe to get rid of bacteria.

MOP UP SHINE Always carry face-blotting papers in your bag. They're handy for late afternoon, when sebum levels peak and your face beams out unwanted shine.

GET FRUITY Look for biological peels and masks that list tropical fruits such as papaya, mango, and pineapple. The enzymes in these fruits will lift loose skin cells clean away without resorting to friction and the irritation that can be a side effect of chemical peels.

JET SET After flying, go to bed wearing a rich moisturizing mask. Don't worry about leaving traces of it on your pillow—your thirsty, oxygen-starved skin will drink it up quickly.

CULTIVATE A BEAUTIFUL MIND Stress tenses up facial muscles, which can lead to a pinched look. Think lovely thoughts, and your face will relax and look serene!

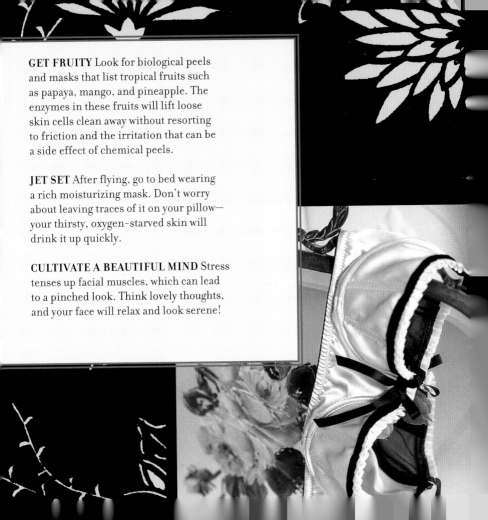

MAKE-
UP

BRIGHT. BEAUTIFUL. FLAWLESS.

When it comes to *catching* someone's eye, it's not always an open-and-shut case of being born *beautiful*; it's about learning how to *bring out* your beauty. And, more often than not, it comes down to the talent of developing a *creative* eye for make-up.

Make-up is and should be fun. After all, it's hardly brain surgery—you can always wipe it off! All too often, we stick to tried-and-tested safe color options, but be *bold* and dare to experiment with new looks. After all, the rewards will be *visible*—your look will be transformed from mundane to *modern*.

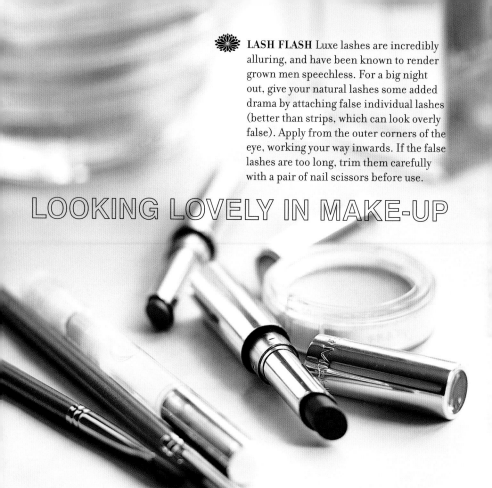

LASH FLASH Luxe lashes are incredibly alluring, and have been known to render grown men speechless. For a big night out, give your natural lashes some added drama by attaching false individual lashes (better than strips, which can look overly false). Apply from the outer corners of the eye, working your way inwards. If the false lashes are too long, trim them carefully with a pair of nail scissors before use.

LOOKING LOVELY IN MAKE-UP

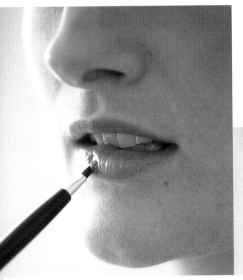

LUXURY LINER For a foolproof smoky eye, take a black, waxy soft pencil and draw a line close along the base of the upper lashes. Get that all-important cat's-eye effect by elongating the line out from the outer corners of the eye. If necessary, lengthen your brow with a pencil to match.

MASCARA MAGIC For the thickest-looking lashes, opt for a fat brush and apply mascara by working the brush close into the roots (tilt your face upwards in the mirror so you can really see them), then flicking the wand outwards towards the tips of the lashes. Look beyond black, too. Deep burgundy mascara, for example, magnifies blue and green eyes marvelously.

GLISTEN UP YOUR SKIN Choose a light fluid foundation rather than a heavy matte one. Too much coverage will not only highlight fine lines and wrinkles, but will also make your skin look overly made-up, which looks aging. Warm the fluid in between clean fingertips, then blend into the skin. To create a subtle gleam, dab a small amount of highlighter fluid along the top of your cheekbones and down the bridge of your nose.

TOE THERAPY Once a month, treat yourself to a pedicure and encourage your pedicurist to go all out on the nail buffing. This will help remove the yellow staining often caused by the dark pigmentation in bright nail polishes.

CARRY A COMPACT It makes powdering your nose just a little bit more glamorous!

SHARPEN UP When using pencils, keep the tip of your lip pencil rounded and soft to prevent a hard and unflattering lip line. Regularly sharpen your eye pencils to keep them pointed. This keeps application precise, helping you get as near to the lash line as possible.

WOW YOUR BROWS For a perfect arch, either book a professional and get them tweezed, waxed, or threaded, or, if you're confident, shape your own. Brush the brows straight up with an eyelash comb and trim straggly hairs with a pair of nail scissors. Next, brush into shape and tidy up the browline by plucking stray hairs from underneath the brow. Use a pair of slanted tweezers for precise plucking. Your brows should start in line with your outer nostril and end above the outer corner of your eye. Don't be tempted to over-pluck—overly skinny brows will give you a look of perpetual surprise!

BE A LOUD MOUTH Red lipstick is a predictable choice for a quick makeover, but it can be a hard color to pull off. It also makes thin lips look thinner. Bold and beautiful-looking lips needn't mean bright: luscious deep pinks, rich chocolates, and berry hues can be just as show-stopping. If you're color-shy, start with a gloss for a hint of color, then graduate to a rich pigmented lipstick. If you're going for look-at-me lips, play down the cheeks. A natural cream cheek tint will give subtle definition.

PICK UP ON PASTELS Don't think pastels are girly—they can look gutsy too. Soft blues, gorgeous greens, and luscious lilacs can really make the eyes pop without looking harsh. Sweep on a sheer layer of shadow all the way up to the brows (for more depth, apply it with a dampened eyeshadow brush), then punch up your look by coating the lashes with a lengthening mascara.

HIDE AWAY BLEMISHES Pimples take time to disguise properly. Rule number one: don't apply cover straight from a concealer stick, as it will look messy and thick, drawing the eye to the area you're trying to conceal. Rule number two: skillfully disguise by using a small, firm brush, loading it up with concealer, and dabbing lightly in the center and around the pimple. Rule number three: blend out until you achieve now-you-see-it, now-you-don't coverage. To conceal well, you need to match your concealer with your skin tone. If you can't find one off the shelf, try mixing two shades for your own customized color.

FRAGRANCE YOUR MOUTH On a romantic dinner date, order a jasmine tea after your meal. It has a delightful aroma (more delicate than mint), so your breath will, too!

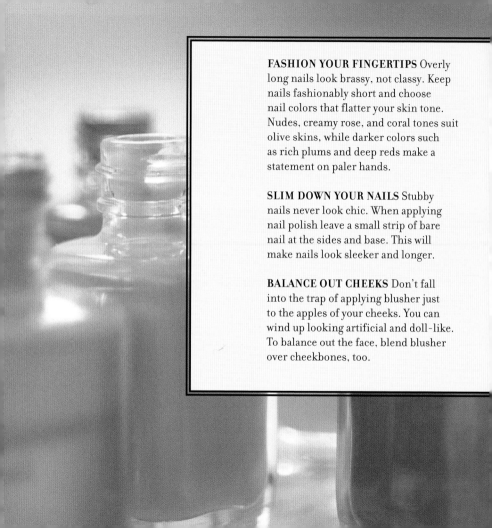

FASHION YOUR FINGERTIPS Overly long nails look brassy, not classy. Keep nails fashionably short and choose nail colors that flatter your skin tone. Nudes, creamy rose, and coral tones suit olive skins, while darker colors such as rich plums and deep reds make a statement on paler hands.

SLIM DOWN YOUR NAILS Stubby nails never look chic. When applying nail polish leave a small strip of bare nail at the sides and base. This will make nails look sleeker and longer.

BALANCE OUT CHEEKS Don't fall into the trap of applying blusher just to the apples of your cheeks. You can wind up looking artificial and doll-like. To balance out the face, blend blusher over cheekbones, too.

GO FOR GOLD If you're stuck in an eyeshadow comfort zone of neutral taupe shades, modernize your look in one easy step by sweeping a golden bronze hue across the lid and underneath the lower lashes. The result? It delivers intensity, so your eyes will mesmerize.

PREP YOUR LIDS Less haste, more preparation is always the key to a better-made-up eye. Always prep your lids first with a dusting of translucent powder to help your eyeshadow stay true, clean-looking, and, most importantly, creaseless throughout the day.

SLICK YOUR BROWS Run a fingertip coated with Vaseline over your eyebrows to bring a dewy, darker shine to them. It's very sexy!

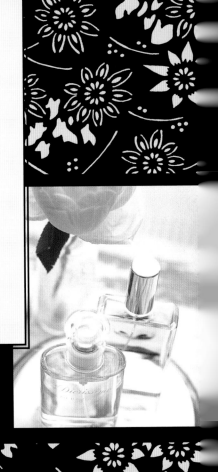

WAKE UP TIRED EYES No amount of eyeshadow can disguise fatigued eyes. Wake up computer-weary peepers by blending a highlighter (keep it in your desk drawer) onto your brow bone and applying concealer to the innermost corner of your eyes. It will magically brighten this shadowy area.

BRONZE AU NATUREL Bronzer can look unnatural and even grubby when applied over your entire face. Limit it to your forehead, the apples of your cheeks, and a little on your nose. An alternative to powder is a liquid bronzer, which gives well-moisturized skin a subtle "I-just-got-back-from-Bali" glow.

SMILE SURGERY Have your teeth professionally whitened. Although it's costly, the results are remarkable. First, you smile more, and second, stain-free teeth make you look healthier, younger, and more desirable.

A MODERN FLUSH Creams and powder aren't the only options for blush. Cheek tints and gels are less intense, as they create a veil of sheer color and a sheer glow. Performing their best on well-moisturized, blemish-free skin, they blend effortlessly and work well with minimal make-up.

TWO HUES IN ONE Keep eyes glamorous by experimenting with duo palettes. Find a color combo that brings out the best in your eye and skin color and wash the brighter hue across the whole of the lid. Now dampen your brush, load it up with the darker shade, and use it to line close to the base of the lashes to ground the look.

SHIMMER FOR SOFTNESS Dab a tiny bit of gold eye shimmer onto the center of your lower lip. It warms up bold lipstick tones and creates a sensual effect.

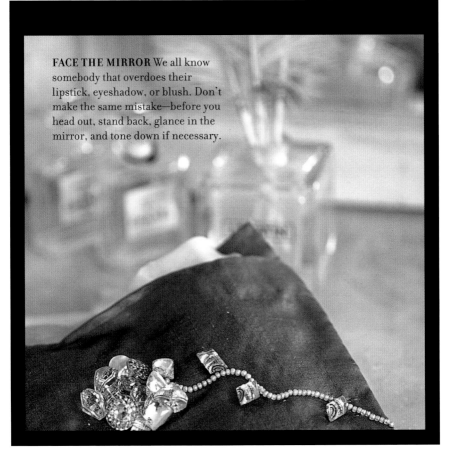

FACE THE MIRROR We all know somebody that overdoes their lipstick, eyeshadow, or blush. Don't make the same mistake—before you head out, stand back, glance in the mirror, and tone down if necessary.

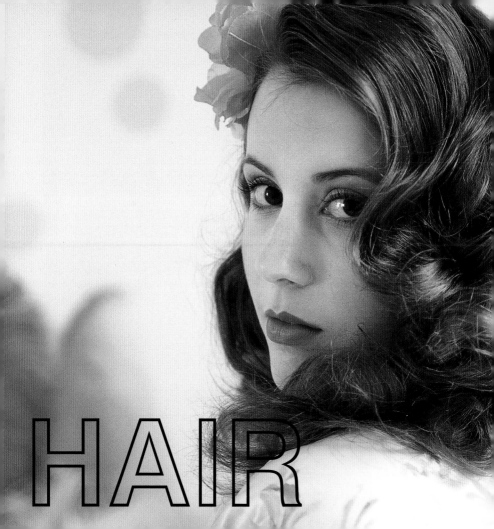

SLEEK. SOPHISTICATED. *DREAMY*.

Far from being an out-of-reach fantasy, the *good* news is that *gorgeous* tresses are well within your grasp. All that is required is a handful of hair tips and the skillful styling *secrets* that top stylists have up their sleeves.

A good haircut can be better than surgery, enhancing cheekbones you never even knew you had. But *amazing* hair doesn't just depend on a *great cut* (although, of course, you should track down a great stylist and put them on speed dial). It's also about having the *confidence* to try different things. A shot of color, for instance, will not only deliver thicker, *richer*-looking hair, but will also make eyes *shine* and skin *glow*. Knowing how to get to grips with the myriad hair products available is equally important. Here's how to get the *heavenly* hair you deserve.

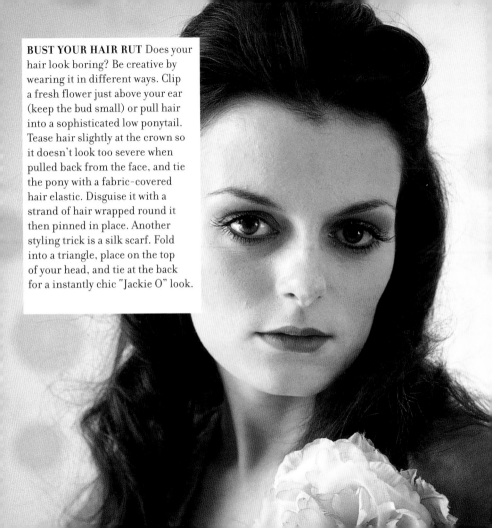

BUST YOUR HAIR RUT Does your hair look boring? Be creative by wearing it in different ways. Clip a fresh flower just above your ear (keep the bud small) or pull hair into a sophisticated low ponytail. Tease hair slightly at the crown so it doesn't look too severe when pulled back from the face, and tie the pony with a fabric-covered hair elastic. Disguise it with a strand of hair wrapped round it then pinned in place. Another styling trick is a silk scarf. Fold into a triangle, place on the top of your head, and tie at the back for a instantly chic "Jackie O" look.

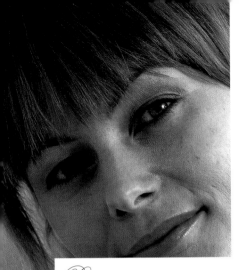

PARTY-PROOF YOUR HAIR When the party heats up, don't let the humidity go to your head. Instead, give your tresses some retro height and backcomb roots with a fine-toothed comb. This hair-saving trick guarantees your locks won't flop!

ℛETHINK YOUR RESTYLE Want to make over your hair, but don't want to lose the length? Be bold and ask your stylist to give you an edgier, more modern version of what you already have. Alternatively, consider bangs. You don't have to go short—bangs that graze your lashes and sweep off to the side will not only vamp up your style, but will also make you look younger!

HEAVENLY HAIR

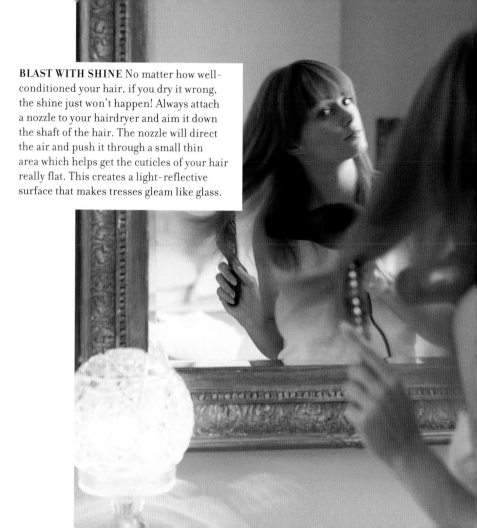

BLAST WITH SHINE No matter how well-conditioned your hair, if you dry it wrong, the shine just won't happen! Always attach a nozzle to your hairdryer and aim it down the shaft of the hair. The nozzle will direct the air and push it through a small thin area which helps get the cuticles of your hair really flat. This creates a light-reflective surface that makes tresses gleam like glass.

DO A DETOX Styling residue build-up results in limp hair. For style queens who rely on products for a well-behaved "do," lather up with a clarifying shampoo once a week to de-gunk and keep your hair squeaky-clean. Now feel the bounce!

SPRAY ON GLOSS Your hair will never be heavenly if you rinse it in the bathwater. It's full of soap and dead skin cells! Always use a detachable shower spray to wash hair, so you can direct the water flow at the roots of the hair and the nape of the neck to ensure a clean sweep.

GROOM ON THE GO For high style on the run, always have a purse-sized paddle brush, a travel tub of serum, and a hair elastic in your bag for on-the-spot taming. Always handy if you've been caught in the rain and the only style rescue is a casual-looking ponytail.

ROLL WITH IT Give oomph to your hair by using large Velcro rollers to create glamorous tousled waves. Take sections of hair and roll each one around a large roller—no pins required. Mist your head lightly with hairspray, relax for 10 minutes, then remove the rollers. Shake out the curls and rake through the hair with fingers. Use a little smoothing wax to tame ends for high glamour.

FIGHT FLUFF If your hair fluffs up after a blowout, swoosh a fine mist of hairspray over the hair. Now use the cold setting on your hairdryer to break up the ends and stop hair looking solid. Finish by running a small amount of serum through the hair to seal cuticles against moisture.

BRUSH UP ON TACTICS Dirty combs and brushes add up to dull-as-ditchwater hair. Shampoo bristles and teeth once a week, and notice how much shinier your hair looks.

HAVE A BLOWOUT Book yourself in for a professional blowout before a night out or just when you want to look your best. It may feel extravagant, but the payback is ready-made glamour and luxurious-looking hair. Make use of the expense by picking up styling tips and techniques while in the capable hands of your stylist.

GLAM UP GRAY Many women confess that one of their biggest beauty challenges is root regrowth before they're ready to hit the salon again. To temporarily disguise offending grey roots on dark hair, coat with a brown or black mascara. For blondes, roots are more obvious, so avert the eye by switching from a straight part to a zigzag parting.

LAYER LESS Take note: the fewer layers in your cut, the sleeker your hair will look, and the greater the shine.

BE WISE—WINTERIZE Central heating can not only be terribly drying to your skin, but also to your hair. Alternate a moisturizing shampoo with your usual shampoo to help re-nourish the hair.

SHADE SMART Don't be tempted to dye your own hair—it will end up saturated in one block color, which will dampen down your complexion. And steer clear of henna. It looks too solid, and even colorists have a problem removing the red tones from the hair. The best-looking dye jobs have two or three toning hues woven through the hair, which only a professional colorist can achieve.

POWER UP Buy the most powerful hairdryer you can find. As a guideline, a salon dryer is a mighty 3,200 watts. It dries hair quicker, and therefore you spend less time damaging your hair.

BE LEAD BY TEXTURE For a head start, when it comes to styling, choose products designed for hair texture, not whether your hair is normal, oily, or dry. These terms generally describe the condition of your scalp, not your hair. Any hair texture can look fabulous, if you know what to style it with.

PRODUCT PROFESSIONAL How you apply styling gel, balm, or wax can make or break your style. The trick is to massage the product into your hands—just like hand cream—then run your hands through your hair. Don't apply too close to the roots, or hair will look greasy.

KNOW YOUR GOOS Serums are best for taming ends of hair, volumizing mousses are designed for roots, and pomades and waxes should be lightly patted over long hair or used to mold short hair.

HONOR YOUR STRAIGHTENING IRONS Straightening irons have become a split-second saviour in the style stakes, but there is little doubt they drink up essential moisture and can put hair on the road to ruin. To prevent such disasters, buy straighteners with ceramic plates, which give hair a little more TLC, use a protection mist, and glide the irons down the hair shaft swiftly. And don't use them every day!

SLEEPING BEAUTY Always brush your hair before hitting your pillow (which should be satin, if possible—it ruffles the hair less than cotton). Brushing not only stimulates the blood circulation, which feeds the roots of the hair, but sets it in place before you lay your head to rest. This will help keep your style intact. In the morning, simply tousle hair with your fingers and give it a quick blast of reviving spray.

TWICE AS NICE Take a tip from your salon and shampoo your hair twice. The first wash breaks down any grease and dirt; the second wash really cleans. Take your time, too—at least three minutes each wash, from first suds to final rinse.

FLIP YOUR HEAD For va-va-voom volume that sees out the day, the easiest trick is a head flip. Blow-dry hair until it's around 80 percent dry, then throw your head upside down. Dry by gently lifting your hair away from the scalp so the heat volumizes the roots. Once hair is dry, flip your head back up and use a smoothing brush to tame it.

DON'T BE FLAKY Snowflakes on your little black dress is so not a good look. A flaky scalp can be brought on by factors such as stress, illness, or a poor diet, so, as well as addressing these, keep your scalp healthy with an Indian head massage. Use olive oil infused with a couple of drops of tea tree and lemon essential oils.

COLOR BOOST Keep your color looking fresh and bright in between salon visits by shampooing with a color glaze. This works especially well for redheads, as their fiery tones fade the quickest.

EAT PROTEIN Hair is protein-hungry (after all, that's what it's made up of), so beautify it from within. Strengthen the hair and guard against hair loss by eating nuts, legumes, fish or lean meat, whole-wheat bread, and vegetables every day. Moisture is important for hair health, so keep your tresses hydrated by drinking plenty of water, and use a rich conditioning mask once a week.

SCENT YOUR CUTICLES Why save fragrance just for your pulse points? Gorgeous hair always smells delicious, so scent with a hair perfume after styling. Alternatively, spritz your signature perfume on your hairbrush and run through from roots to tips. Your hair will subtly exude your fragrance as you move your head from side to side.

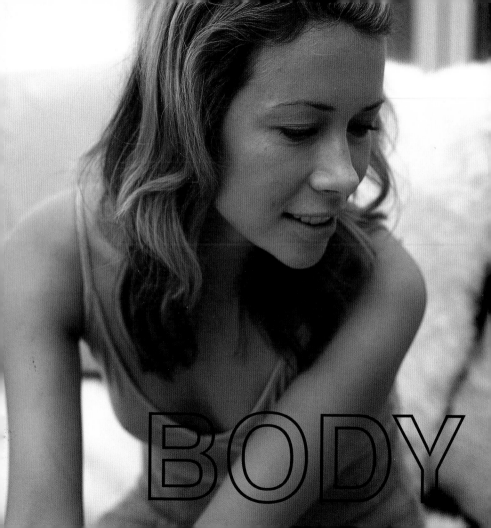

BODY

STRONG. HEALTHY. *B*EAUTIFUL.

Having the body beautiful doesn't depend on your dress size: it comes from the *confidence* of being happy in your own skin, whatever your shape. If a size tag makes you feel a failure, snip it out when you get home! A survey revealed that millions of women would pay thousands of dollars of their hard-earned cash for the *perfect* body, but cosmetic surgery isn't the only way to a shapelier, smoother, more *gorgeous-looking* body.

Your body is a *hot* accessory and how you treat it, think about it, and wear it can make all the difference to how you *feel* about yourself. Finding your inner *goddess* isn't hard—you just need lots of *positive* thought, a little pampering, and the determination to keep your body *fit* and running smoothly. That's the key to feeling gorgeous—both in and out of your clothes.

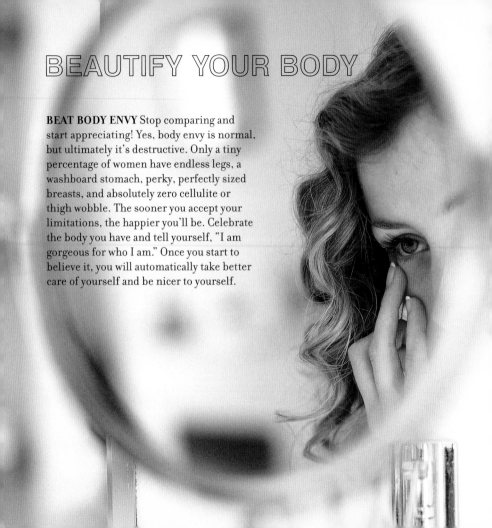

BEAUTIFY YOUR BODY

BEAT BODY ENVY Stop comparing and start appreciating! Yes, body envy is normal, but ultimately it's destructive. Only a tiny percentage of women have endless legs, a washboard stomach, perky, perfectly sized breasts, and absolutely zero cellulite or thigh wobble. The sooner you accept your limitations, the happier you'll be. Celebrate the body you have and tell yourself, "I am gorgeous for who I am." Once you start to believe it, you will automatically take better care of yourself and be nicer to yourself.

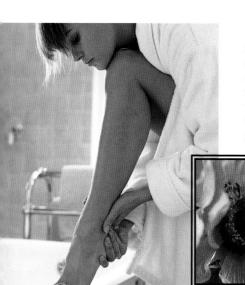

SPICE GIRL Improve oxygenation and skin tone by opting for a body scrub containing ginger. It will warm the skin to increase the flow of oxygen to the skin's surface, remove dead skin cells, and stimulate new cell growth for a gorgeous glow.

SOLE SURVIVOR Nothing looks less elegant than a woman who hobbles, limps, or shuffles. Visit a podiatrist to tackle any painful corns or bunions brought on by tight shoes or sky-high stilettos. Once your feet are dealt with, your wrinkles will relax, too. Pain always shows on your face first!

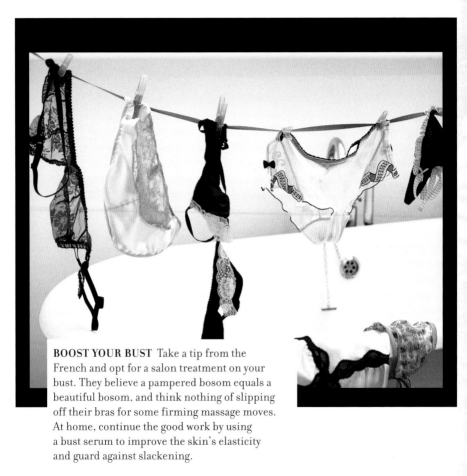

BOOST YOUR BUST Take a tip from the French and opt for a salon treatment on your bust. They believe a pampered bosom equals a beautiful bosom, and think nothing of slipping off their bras for some firming massage moves. At home, continue the good work by using a bust serum to improve the skin's elasticity and guard against slackening.

WALK SLOWLY Stop rushing and Take. Your. Time... even if it means leaving 10 minutes early to get to your destination on time. Strolling in a leisurely fashion is sexy and attracts admiring glances. Put a little runway action into your stroll, too. Tilt your shoulders back and push your chest forward. And, unlike power-walking, where the arms are used as pistons, let them trail slightly behind your frame.

GYM 'N' TONIC Join a gym which has a great pool, a large steam room, and a juice bar. It makes pounding the treadmill all the more bearable if there's something to look forward to post-exercise!

DIM THE LIGHTS When naked, don't willingly spotlight your flaws. Fill the bedroom with tiny votives, so your body is lit with flattering, amber-hued candlelight.

GET PERSONAL Whether you want to be firmer, leaner, or stronger, get into shape by calling in the services of a personal trainer. Why not share the sessions with a girlfriend? It cuts the cost, introduces an element of friendly competition, and keeps up motivation levels.

SEE OFF BACNE If you're susceptible to a pimply back, a change of routine may be all that's needed. When showering, lather and rinse your hair before you wash your body. When hair conditioners or masks are washed out, they can leave a fine film on the back that results in blocked pores. Shower and cleanse post-shampooing, and you will automatically rinse off any pimple-producing residue.

LACE THE WATER Never take a bath leaving the water naked. It's a beauty sin! Always add something: bubbles, salts, oils, or petals. Bathing should be a mini-luxury slipped in at the end of the day.

BOOK A MASSAGE Touch helps you feel comfortable in your own skin. Don't feel embarrassed about your body, either. It reflects your life—from scars to stretchmarks—and it's a part of what makes you individual. Seek out massages beyond the gentle aromatherapy version. A sports massage benefits not only athletes, but anyone who walks in heels and totes a heavy shoulder bag every day of the week. A Thai massage will stretch the mind as well as the body with its combination of Swedish massage techniques and yogalike stretches. It's one of the best ways to simultaneously bliss out and tone up.

WAX WORKS It's the only depilatory that will give legs a beautiful sheen. When waxing at home, lightly dust the area to be waxed with talcum powder. This will absorb any oil on the skin, giving the wax a better grip. Post-waxing, avoid hot baths and sunbathing, to allow the skin to settle.

VEIN HOPES Thread veins can blight an otherwise great-looking pair of legs. Look for leg creams with vitamin K (used to clot leaking blood vessels) or consider laser therapy or sclerotherapy. The former involves targeting and zapping veins, while the latter involves injecting a saline solution into the offending vein, which will then collapse and hopefully vanish. Just make sure you get it done long before heading off on vacation, as the injection area can be left bruised and swollen.

FUSE YOUR FITNESS Beat body boredom with fusion fitness. By addressing the yin and yang of exercise, you will not only balance out your body but your mind, too. Interspersing aerobic workouts with yoga classes, for instance, will have the benefits of burning fat and stretching and toning your muscles, then downloading your brain and blessing you with a Zenlike calm.

SEE YOU LATER, CELLULITE

There's nothing like instant results to boost your resolve to stick to regular exercise and a good eating plan. Treat yourself to one of the new generation of cellulite treatments to give orange-peel thighs a good working over. Carry the good efforts on at home with lifting and gentle pinching massage movements to enhance muscle tone and stimulate circulation and lymph flow.

RAISE YOUR FEET

Every evening, take 10 minutes out to pile up the pillows and raise your feet higher than your head. Not only does it literally take the weight off your feet, it also guards against swollen ankles and varicose veins. If you have time, improve your circulation by massaging with a reviving blend of essential oils. Mix two drops each of rosemary, lavender, and juniper into 3 tablespoons of almond oil. Using firm movements, massage into the calves and down the front of the legs.

STRETCH AND LENGTHEN

At the end of a stressful day you will often find that you are shorter than you were at the start of the day. To ease out hunched shoulders, try this simple move to get your upper back mobile and bring you back up to your real height. It's a perfect exercise to take you from desk to dance floor. Roll up a medium-sized towel so it makes a sausage about 4 inches wide. Lie on your back with it under your bra strap for about 10 minutes, and during this time extend your arms over your head several times. This will stretch the spinal ligaments that pull your upper back forward.

SUCK IN YOUR TUMMY

No matter what you are doing, consciously draw your navel back towards your spine. This not only helps activate the core muscles that protect your spine (your body's inner corset), but helps improve your posture and works towards giving you a flatter tummy.

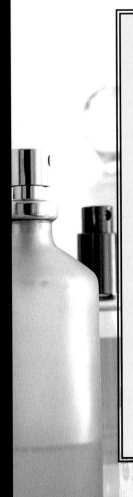

GLIMMER SKIN Make skin tone vibrant by adding shimmer. Powders, lotions, and highlighting sticks that boast a small amount of iridescent shimmer spotlight the skin by reflecting light and throwing the area into soft focus. It's a little like having your own lighting technician! Satinize and slenderize your limbs by applying shimmer down the center of legs, then across the collarbones, along the shoulders, and in between the breasts.

DRESS UP YOUR BATHROOM Buy body creams in beautiful and unusual jars. It's a way of bringing dressing-table decadence into your bathroom and making you feel absolutely gorgeous. Always try to moisturize within a minute of bathing or showering. This way, the cream traps much-needed moisture from the water, guaranteeing silky-soft skin.

WEIGHTS-TO-GO Buy a small set of dumbbells in your favourite color and leave them where you can see them. Whenever you have a spare five minutes, take them in hand and do some arm exercises to firm flabby upper arms.

FOOLPROOF YOUR (FAKE) TAN When looking for sunless color, always work from your toes upwards, as this will avoid telltale creases and smudges brought on from constantly bending over. Alternatively, consider a professional spray tan for a seamless finish. You can even request artistic "shading" to give your stomach and breasts added definition. Don't forget—always use a separate self-tanner for your face, as it will contain less oil than a tanner formulated for the body.

STRIKE A POSE Don't stand with your arms folded. It looks matronly, crumples your posture, and does nothing for your sensuality factor. Instead, stand with a hand lightly resting on an exaggerated hip. This simple move oozes confidence, creates a womanly curve and shows off your figure to best advantage.

ASK FOR COMPLIMENTS Go on: ask your man what he loves about your body! And ask him to repeat it often—especially when making love. He will be more than happy to oblige and it will make you feel fabulous about yourself.

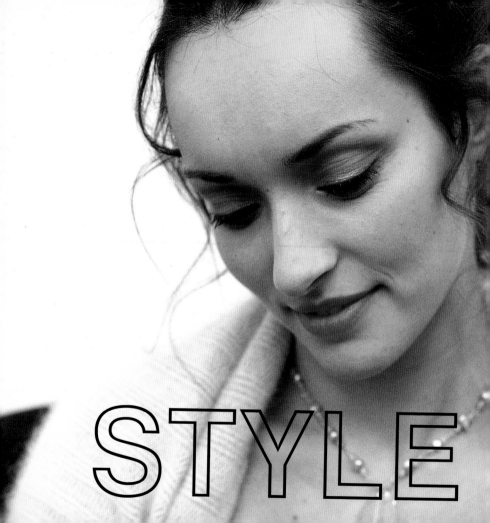

COOL. CONFIDENT. *CHIC*.

Every woman knows that if you feel *good* in what you're wearing,
you'll instantly *stand out* when you stroll into a room.
Stand-out *style* doesn't even have to be all glitz and *glam*.
A dress-down outfit can be just as *chic*—it's just making sure
the T-shirt is the right shape, and that your jeans fit properly
to create the effect of a nice pert bottom!

Dressing well and looking *stylish* has never been so easy.
With racks of designer-inspired threads in the stores, you
don't need to spend a fortune to look *fabulous*. Everyday glamour is
not hard to achieve; it's about being *imaginative* with accessories
and choosing clothes that bless you with that certain "X" factor.
Ultimately, *feeling* fabulous in clothes comes down to that
old saying: it's not what you wear, it's how you wear it.

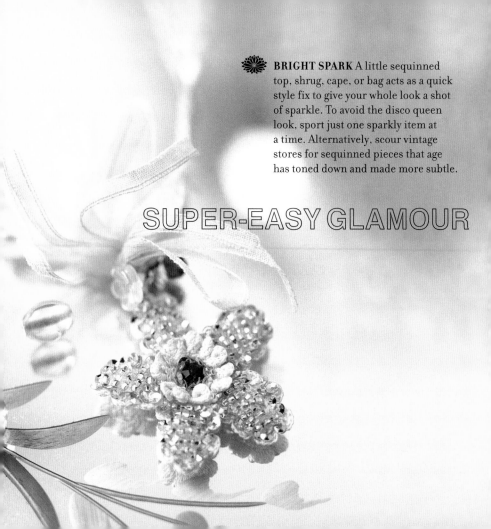

BRIGHT SPARK A little sequinned top, shrug, cape, or bag acts as a quick style fix to give your whole look a shot of sparkle. To avoid the disco queen look, sport just one sparkly item at a time. Alternatively, scour vintage stores for sequinned pieces that age has toned down and made more subtle.

SUPER-EASY GLAMOUR

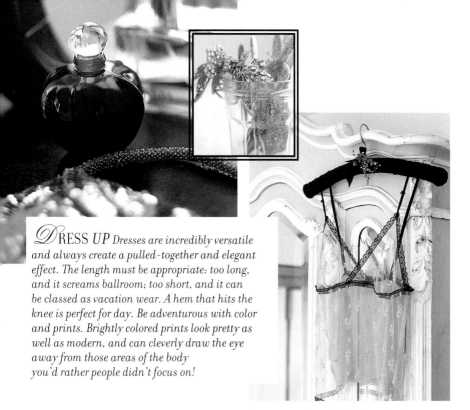

*D*RESS UP *Dresses are incredibly versatile and always create a pulled-together and elegant effect. The length must be appropriate: too long, and it screams ballroom; too short, and it can be classed as vacation wear. A hem that hits the knee is perfect for day. Be adventurous with color and prints. Brightly colored prints look pretty as well as modern, and can cleverly draw the eye away from those areas of the body you'd rather people didn't focus on!*

Luxe easy pieces A basic camisole top can look less boring in chiffon or silk. Look for fabrics that have a "voice" rather than staying mute.

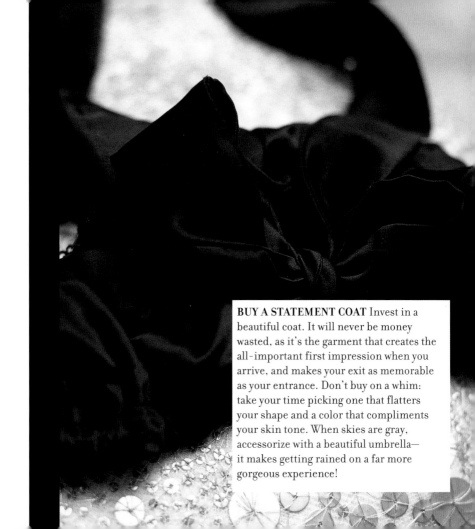

BUY A STATEMENT COAT Invest in a beautiful coat. It will never be money wasted, as it's the garment that creates the all-important first impression when you arrive, and makes your exit as memorable as your entrance. Don't buy on a whim: take your time picking one that flatters your shape and a color that compliments your skin tone. When skies are gray, accessorize with a beautiful umbrella— it makes getting rained on a far more gorgeous experience!

LUXE LEISUREWEAR

Downtime clothes shouldn't look down and out, so dump those shapeless leggings now! For chilling out at home, opt for silky pajama bottoms teamed with a slinky T-shirt. Alternatively, if you prefer a starlet effect, opt for boudoir chic and slink around in a silk cami under a kimono-style gown.

WEAR WHITES ONCE Never wear anything white twice. Whether it be a shirt, pants, or a T-shirt, wear it only once before washing. White needs to look spotless, not stale.

CARDIGAN CHIC Cardigans aren't just for the twinset-and-pearls set—they can really add to your outfit and make chic cover-ups. Choose slim-fitting knits in bright colors and layer them over T-shirts, dresses, and shirts. If you can, save up and buy cashmere—it will make you feel like a millionairess!

LIFT, DON'T SQUISH Bras that boost don't always make your breasts look their best. They can end up looking squashed. Try a balconette bra for a smooth uplift. Choose bras with pretty colored or decorated straps, too—they encourage you to enjoy your underwear, and make a big difference when on show.

MIX 'N' MATCH An overly co-ordinated look can give the effect you've stepped straight out of a catalogue. Inject your own signature style by mixing old with new—a smart sweater with a pair of faded jeans, or a savvy pair of smart slacks and a luxury jacket teamed with a pair of colorful sneakers.

BELT UP If you've got a wasp waist, give it star billing and cinch it in with a wide belt. As well as adding a dash of French chic, a belt will create definition and pull separates together in high style.

SUPERSIZE SHADES The glamorous and the fabulous always wear oversized shades. Not only do they lend a VIP vibe, but they're also the ideal cover-up for fatigued eyes.

LOVE LAYERS Experimenting with layers—short sleeves worn over long; dresses worn over jeans—liberates and funks up your look. The only rule? Just check that your overall proportions balance out your figure.

TRY MENSWEAR A slouchy boyfriend cut can look surprisingly sexy and feminine. Generously cut pants and vests add a dash of *Annie Hall* cool when twinned with high heels and delicate shirts.

FRAME YOUR FACE A beautiful jeweled necklace or a pair of sparkly earrings will reflect light onto your face and instantly pretty up your complexion.

ORGANIZE YOUR WARDROBE It's one of the first steps to style. Weed out any items you haven't worn for a year. Then color-code your outfits—it's easier to see what you've got, and more inspiring. Sort your shoe pile and put them into pairs. Finally, do a quick clothes inspection. Secure any loose buttons, de-fluff with a sticky roller, and hang garments on padded satin hangers. Not only will they bring a touch of class to your closet, but they also keep clothes in better shape.

SPANGLE UP YOUR SWEATER A plain-knit crew neck is the perfect canvas for a bold necklace. It's a fantastic way to introduce grown-up glamour to a daytime look.

FLASH SOME FLESH But not too much! A hint of décolletage or baring one shoulder keeps your look sexy, seductive, and modern.

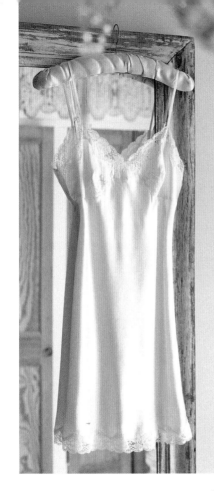

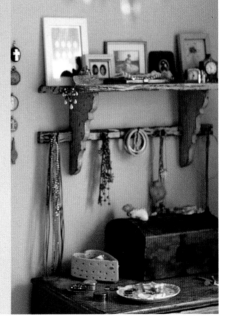

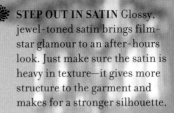 **STEP OUT IN SATIN** Glossy, jewel-toned satin brings film-star glamour to an after-hours look. Just make sure the satin is heavy in texture—it gives more structure to the garment and makes for a stronger silhouette.

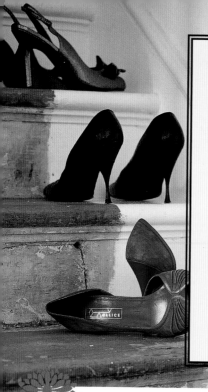

WEAR WEDGES If you can't wear heels, try wedges instead. They give the height without the wobble, and are sexy and fun to wear with dresses.

LENGTHEN THOSE LEGS Add inches to your height—wear straight-legged jeans extra long and team them with high heels.

DON'T HIDE Baggy clothes don't hide anything: in fact, they make you look bigger. Dress to show off your curves instead.

GO LONG ON EARRINGS Make earrings noticeable and dramatic by wearing them long. Showcase them by sweeping hair away from your neck.

LEARN TO GLIDE The most expensive of heels will never look elegant if you stamp. Shorten your stride and take baby steps, making sure you put the heel down first and then slide. If all else fails, downsize to a smaller heel!

LIFE'S RICH TAPESTRY When on vacation overseas, always keep your eyes open for interesting fashion finds. Often you can pick up unusual prints, fabrics, and designs you would never find at home. This way, you're buying something original, unique, and one-of-a-kind.

WATCH MOVIES Who needs front-row tickets to the Paris shows when you can bring a fashion extravaganza into your own sitting room? Faye Dunaway brought a whole new meaning to wearing a beret in *Bonnie and Clyde*, while Marilyn Monroe exudes classic Hollywood glamour in *Some Like it Hot*. In *Butterfield 8*, Elizabeth Taylor makes every woman want to upgrade her lingerie drawer immediately, and, for those that like polished glitz, check out Sharon Stone in *Casino*.

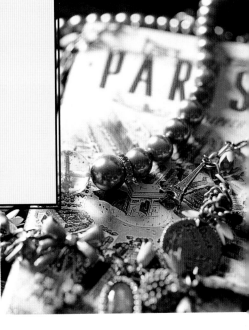

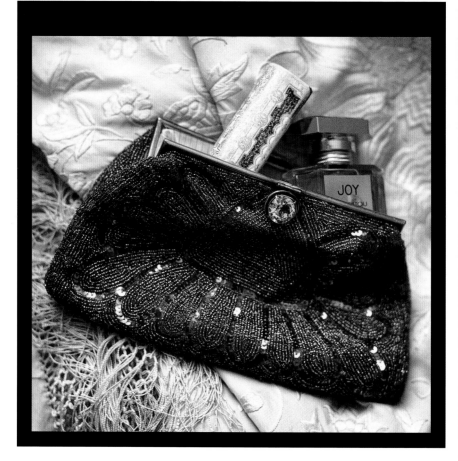

HANDBAG HABITS Don't carry the same purse day in, day out. Change them constantly, as you would an outfit. When shopping, try them on for size, too. If you're small, huge totes can make you look dumpy. And if you're tall, tiny bags can make you look huge. Vintage bags are a great buy, as the leather looks tactile and slouchy rather than stiff and new.

HAND CANDY Make a bold fashion statement by slipping on a large and opulent cocktail ring. It will glam up any outfit and does for the hands what polish does for the nails.

FUNKY FLATS Never feel that flat shoes should be plain. Compensate for the lack of a look-at-me heel by going for shiny, metallic, or bejeweled styles. Wear with Audrey Hepburn-style cigarette pants or neat little A-line skirts.

HOLD A CLUTCH There's something about a clutch that always makes a woman feel sophisticated and feminine. It also has the habit of keeping your figure looking streamlined. Seek out purses with interesting detail such as beads, and those with sumptuous textures such as grosgrain, velvet, or satin.

FLIP OUT Don't routinely think party dresses require high heels. When wearing a long evening dress, slip a pair of fabulous sparkly flip-flops onto perfectly pedicured feet. It's a stylish compromise between being dressed up (for glamour) and dressed down (for comfort).

BE BOOTYLICIOUS Boots equal seduction. When a great pair of boots are pulled on, a woman will not merely stroll, but stride. Boots are led by fashion trends, so are best updated each winter, or at least every other year.

useful addresses

NUTRITION & FITNESS

Fitness Together
www.fitnesstogether.com
Personal-training studios located
nationwide. You'll receive one-
on-one fitness instruction and
a program will be designed to
suit your specific needs.

InVite Health
800-844-9060
www.invitehealth.com
Nutritional boutiques in the New
York metro area. Accredited
nutritionists offer free health-
and diet-related advice.

**American Massage Therapy
Association**
500 Davis Street,
Suite 900
Evanston, IL 60201
847 864 0123
www.amtamassage.org
Help with finding a massage
therapist near you.

Yoga
www.yogafinder.com
Links to yoga teachers, workshops,
and retreats.

SKINCARE

Aveda
Call 866 823 1425 or visit
www.aveda.com for your nearest
retailer.
Eco-friendly skin- and haircare.

**American Academy of
Dermatology**
Call 888-462-DERM or visit
www.aad.org to find a
dermatologist in your area through
the site's extensive network of
physicians.

Clarins
Visit www.clarins.com for details
of your nearest retailer.
Skincare products, facial
treatments, and skincare advice.

Philosophy
Call 800-568-3151 or visit
www.philosophy.com for details of
your nearest retailer.
Products that draw on the best of
current medically based skincare
technology. Their specialty is
treating dysfunctional skin
conditions.

EYEBROWS

Anastasia Beverly Hills
www.anastasia.net
Eyebrow guru Anastasia Soare
counts Madonna and Jennifer
Lopez among her clients. Brow
waxing, tweezing, and tinting are
available at her two salons in
California as well as select
Nordstrom and Sephora stores.

Natasha Style & Cut
2759 West Devon Avenue
Chicago, IL 60659
773-761-2274
Salon owner Bharati Nakum is
well-known for her threading
technique, an ancient form of
eyebrow shaping.

HAIR AND MAKEUP

Benefit
Call 800-781-2336 or visit
www.benefitcosmetics.com for
details of your nearest retailer.
Check out the brand's "Fake-it"
collection to help you get gorgeous.

Bobbi Brown
Call 877-310-9222 or visit
www.bobbibrowncosmetics.com
for details of your nearest retailer.

Bobbi Brown counters offer a free personalized makeup lesson.

Estée Lauder

Call 877-311-3883 or visit www.esteelauder.com for details of your nearest retailer

Visit the website to set up a consultation with a beauty advisor at an Estée Lauder counter.

Lips & Locks

642 A. Venice Blvd.
Venice, CA 90291
310-301-8086
www.lipsandlocks.com
A hair and makeup studio helmed by celebrity stylist Sheree Pouls.

Regis Hair Salons

Visit www.regishairstylists.com for details of your nearest salon. Reliable chain of good-value hair salons.

PAMPERING AND TANNING

Canyon Ranch SpaClubs

At The Venetian
3355 Las Vegas Boulevard South,
Suite 1159
Las Vegas, NV 89109
877-220-2688
and
At the Gaylord Palms Resort & Convention Center

6000 W. Osceola Parkway
Kissimmee, FL 34746
407-586-2051
www.canyonranch.com
Hair and makeup, manicures, pedicures, massages, facials, wraps, and body scrubs.

Fantasy Tan

Call 888-FAN-TANS or visit www.fantasytan.com for details of your nearest salon.
Airbrush and spray tans.

mobileSPA

800-651-4740
www.mobilespa.com
Spa services and themed spa parties at home.

Mystic Tan

Visit www.mystictan.com for details of your nearest salon. Get a streakfree sunless tan in their automated mist-on tan booths.

Red Mountain Spa

1275 E. Red Mountain Circle
Ivins, UT 84738
800-407-3002
www.redmountainspa.com
Pampering spa-vacation packages will glamorize you from head to toe.

SPARTY!

646-736-1777
www.spa-party.com
Spa services and parties at home. Available in major metropolitan areas.

St. Tropez Tanning

Call 661-775-6900 or visit www.sttropeztan.com for details of your nearest salon.
The original fake-tan experts.

FRAGRANCE

Diptyque

171 Maiden Lane
San Francisco
CA 94108
415-402-0600
www.diptyqueparis.com
Cult French perfumes for the body and the home. Visit their website for details of their Boston store.

The Fragrance Shop Perfumery

612 Lincoln Road
Miami Beach, FL 33139
305-535-0037
www.thefragranceshop.com
Pure perfume oils inspired by designer fragrances, in addition to a range of house blends.

Sephora
2103 Broadway
New York, NY 10023
212 362 1500
Visit www.sephora.com for
details of your nearest store.
Wide choice of classic and
modern fragrances.

LINGERIE

Agent Provocateur
www.agentprovocateur.com
Saucy little numbers that are
almost too good to hide under
clothes!

La Petite Coquette
888-473-5799
www.thelittleflirt.net
A boudoir-style boutique full
of gorgeous lingerie online.

Victoria's Secret
Call 800-411-5116 or visit
www.victoriassecret.com for
details of your nearest store.
Nationwide chain offering a
variety of seamless, strapless,
and push-up bras that will help
you look fabulous whatever
you're wearing over the top.

JEWELRY

Alex and Ani
www.alexandani.com
Funky jewelry designed for the
21st-century girl.

C.H.A.R.M.
www.charmco.com
Striking antique and vintage-
inspired charms. Many popular
themes—the cute beauty and
fashion charms include a gold
stiletto heel, a credit card, and
even a tiny hairdryer!

Helen Ficalora
www.helenficalora.com
Simple, elegant gold discs
stamped with the letters of the
alphabet and words such as
"love" and "smile."

Tiffany
www.tiffany.com
Classic investment pieces
in gold and silver.

credits

Key: ph. = photographer; a = above;
b = below; l = left; c = center; r = right.

Images taken from *Japanese Patterns*,
published by The Pepin Press
(www.pepinpress.com): 1; 2-3; 5; 6-
7; 12-13 background; 14; 17; 19
background; 24-25; 27 background;
28; 35 – 37; 39 background; 45 – 47;
49; 55 – 56; 61.

Ph. Caroline Arber: 15/designed
and made by Jane Cassini and Ann
Brownfield
(jane_vintagestyle@yahoo.com) 29.

Ph. Dan Duchars: 11 l; 22; 26; 42.

Ph. Daniel Farmer: 33 l; 34; 43 l.

Ph. Winfried Heinze: 11 r; 23 l.

Ph. Sandra Lane: 58 -59.

Ph. David Montgomery: 38; 43 r; 48.

Ph. Claire Richardson: 4; 8; 10; 11c;
18; 19 inset; 23 r; 27 inset; 30; 31; 33
r; 39 inset; 40; 44; 50; 52 53 l; 53 r;
54; 57; 60.

Ph. Pia Tryde: 12 inset.

Ph. Polly Wreford: 43 c; /Foster
House at www.beachstudios.co.uk
16; 53 c.